A Bodyweight Training Guide For Beginners And Seniors

A Step-By-Step Guide To Kegel Exercises; Boosting Strength Gains 7times And Tips For Muscle Building And Achieving Bodybuilding Goals With An Ultimate Diet Plan

Maritza Mitchell

Table of Contents

CHAPTER ONE

Introduction

Kegel exercises, also known as pelvic floor exercises, are designed to strengthen the pelvic floor muscles. These muscles support the bladder, uterus, small intestine, and rectum. Engaging in Kegel exercises can benefit both men and women by improving bladder control, enhancing sexual function, and supporting pelvic organ health.

Step-by-step guide on how to perform Kegel exercises

Identify the Right Muscles: To start, you need to identify your pelvic floor muscles. The easiest way to do this is by stopping your urine flow midstream. However, it's important not to make a habit of stopping urination frequently as this can lead to issues. This action helps you locate the muscles but should not be part of the regular exercise routine.

Find a Comfortable Position: You can perform Kegel exercises in various positions, such as lying down, sitting, or standing. Choose a position that is comfortable for you.

Contract Your Pelvic Floor Muscles: Once you've identified the correct muscles, contract them. It should feel like you're squeezing and lifting the muscles in your pelvic area. Make sure to breathe normally during the exercise and avoid tensing other muscles, like those in your abdomen, thighs, or buttocks.

Hold and Release: Hold the contraction for about 3-5 seconds initially, and then relax for an equal amount of time. Gradually increase the duration of the contractions as your muscles get stronger.

Repeat Regularly: Aim for at least three sets of 10 repetitions per day. You can increase this number as your muscles become stronger.

The Role of Pelvic Floor Muscles

The pelvic floor muscles play a crucial role in supporting the organs in the pelvis, including the bladder, uterus, small intestine, and rectum. These muscles act like a hammock, providing support to these organs and helping maintain their proper position within the pelvis.

Here are some key functions of the pelvic floor muscles:

Supporting Organs: The pelvic floor muscles help support the bladder, uterus, and other pelvic organs, preventing them from prolapsing or descending into the vaginal or rectal areas.

Controlling Urinary and Fecal Function: Strong pelvic floor muscles aid in controlling the release of urine and feces. They help maintain continence by contracting to prevent unwanted leakage and relaxing to allow the release of urine or feces when appropriate.

Enhancing Sexual Function: These muscles play a role in sexual function by contributing to arousal and orgasm. Strong pelvic floor muscles can improve sensations during intercourse for both men and women.

Benefits of strengthening these muscles

Improved Bladder Control: Strengthening the pelvic floor can help reduce or eliminate urinary incontinence, a common issue among both men and women, particularly after childbirth or with age.

Better Bowel Control: Strong pelvic floor muscles contribute to better control over bowel movements, reducing the risk of fecal incontinence.

Enhanced Sexual Health: For both men and women, stronger pelvic floor muscles can lead to improved sexual sensations, increased arousal, and better control over orgasms.

Prevention of Prolapse: Strengthening these muscles can reduce the risk of pelvic organ prolapse, where organs like the bladder, uterus, or rectum descend into the vaginal or rectal areas due to weakened support.

Postnatal Recovery: Women who strengthen their pelvic floor muscles during and after pregnancy can aid in postnatal recovery, helping to regain bladder control and pelvic strength.

Regularly practicing Kegel exercises or other pelvic floor workouts can help individuals strengthen these muscles and reap these benefits. However, it's essential to perform exercises correctly and consistently to see improvements.

Identifying and Engaging Pelvic Floor Muscles

Getting started with Kegel exercises involves identifying and engaging the pelvic floor muscles correctly, along with maintaining proper form and technique. A step-by-step guide to help you get started:

Locate the Muscles: The pelvic floor muscles are the ones you use to stop the flow of urine midstream. However, it's crucial not to make a habit of doing this regularly, as it can lead to issues with bladder emptying.

Alternative Method: Another way to identify these muscles is by imagining you're trying to stop passing gas or trying to tighten the muscles around your vagina or rectum.

CHAPTER TWO

Proper Form and Technique

Find a Comfortable Position: Choose a comfortable position to perform Kegel exercises. You can try lying down, sitting, or standing.

Relax First: Before starting the exercises, take a few deep breaths and relax your body.

Engage the Muscles: Contract your pelvic floor muscles. Imagine pulling the muscles up and in, as if trying to lift them towards your abdomen. Be careful not to tighten your abdominal, buttock, or thigh muscles while doing this.

Hold and Release: Hold the contraction for about 3-5 seconds initially. Gradually work your way up to holding for 10 seconds, if possible. Then, relax for an equal duration.

Repeat Regularly: Aim for at least three sets of 10 repetitions per day. As your muscles get stronger, you can gradually increase the number of sets and repetitions.

Tips for Better Results

Consistency is Key: Perform Kegel exercises regularly for optimal results. Set a schedule or incorporate them into your daily routine.

Avoid Overdoing It: Don't overwork your pelvic floor muscles. Doing too many Kegels or holding them for too long can strain the muscles.

Be Patient: It takes time to see improvements. Stick to the routine and be patient with your progress.

Gradual Advancements and Challenges

Advancing in Kegel exercises involves gradually increasing the challenge level and incorporating advanced techniques to further strengthen the pelvic floor muscles. Here's how you can progress in your Kegel routine:

Increase Duration: Start by gradually increasing the duration of each contraction. Begin with shorter holds (3-5 seconds) and progressively work your way up to longer holds (10 seconds or more) as your muscles become stronger.

Vary Repetitions: Gradually increase the number of repetitions and sets you perform each day. For example, start with three sets of 10 repetitions and gradually add more sets or repetitions over time.

Change Positions: Experiment with different positions while doing Kegel exercises. For instance, try performing them while standing, sitting, or even during specific activities like walking or yoga poses to challenge your muscles in different ways.

Resistance Training: Consider using resistance tools designed for pelvic floor exercises, such as weighted vaginal cones or Kegel balls. These add resistance and challenge your muscles to work harder.

Quick Contractions: Introduce quick and rapid contractions of the pelvic floor muscles. Contract and release the muscles rapidly, aiming for multiple short contractions in quick succession.

Advanced Techniques for Strength

Elevated Positions: Experiment with exercises in elevated positions. For instance, try elevating your hips using a yoga block or performing bridges while engaging your pelvic floor muscles to add intensity.

Integrated Movements: Combine pelvic floor exercises with other movements. For instance, perform squats or lunges while engaging your pelvic floor muscles to integrate the workout and challenge your muscles further.

Breath Coordination: Coordinate your breathing with Kegel exercises. Inhale as you relax your pelvic floor muscles and exhale as you contract them. This synchronization can enhance muscle engagement.

Biofeedback Devices: Use biofeedback devices or apps that provide real-time feedback on muscle contractions. They can help you monitor and optimize your technique for maximum effectiveness.

Advanced Exercise Programs: Consider joining specialized pelvic floor exercise programs or classes led by experts, especially if you're looking for more advanced routines tailored to your needs.

Integrating Kegels into Daily Life

Integrating Kegel exercises into your daily routine can help make them a regular habit. One can establish a Kegel routine and incorporate these exercises into your everyday activities by:

Set Reminders: Use reminders on your phone, calendar, or a dedicated app to prompt you to do Kegel exercises at specific times during the day. Consistency is key, so establish a routine that works for you, whether it's in the morning, during breaks, or before bed.

Pair with Daily Habits: Link Kegel exercises with other daily activities. For example, do a set of exercises while brushing your teeth, waiting in line, or during specific breaks at work.

Create a Visual Cue: Place visual reminders, like sticky notes or cues in your environment, to prompt you to perform your Kegels. This could be a note on your bathroom mirror or on your desk.

Track Progress: Keep a Kegel exercise log or use an app to track your progress. Monitoring your routine and progress can motivate you to stay consistent.

CHAPTER THREE
Incorporating Kegels in Everyday Activities

During Commutes: Practice Kegels while commuting—whether driving, riding the bus, or sitting on a train. It's a discreet way to work on pelvic floor strength during your daily travel.

While Watching TV or Reading: Use TV commercial breaks or reading intervals as cues to perform a set of Kegel exercises. This can turn passive moments into opportunities for strengthening.

At Work: Incorporate Kegel exercises into your work routine. Set reminders to do a set every hour or during specific breaks. You can discreetly perform these exercises while seated.

During Physical Activities: Engage your pelvic floor muscles during physical activities like walking, running, or doing yoga poses. It can enhance the effectiveness of the exercises.

Household Chores: Connect Kegel exercises with household chores. For example, do a set while doing dishes, folding laundry, or cooking.

Tips for Success

Be Consistent: Consistency is key to seeing progress. Stick to your routine even if you're doing just a few sets at a time.

Make it a Habit: Associate Kegel exercises with specific triggers or activities to create a habit loop that reinforces the routine.

Be Patient: Results take time. Be patient and persistent with your routine to see improvements in pelvic floor strength.

Kegels during Pregnancy and Postpartum

Kegel exercises have specific considerations for both pregnancy/postpartum and men's health:

During Pregnancy: Kegel exercises can benefit pregnant individuals by strengthening pelvic floor muscles, potentially easing delivery and aiding in postnatal recovery. However, it's crucial to consult a healthcare professional before starting any new exercise routine during pregnancy.

Postpartum Recovery: After childbirth, Kegel exercises can help in toning and re-strengthening pelvic floor muscles. These exercises may assist in regaining bladder control and addressing issues like urinary incontinence that might arise after childbirth.

Proper Technique: It's essential for pregnant individuals and those in the postpartum phase to perform Kegels correctly. Overexertion or incorrect technique could potentially cause more harm than good. Consulting a pelvic floor physical therapist for guidance on proper technique is highly recommended.

Postnatal Guidance: Engaging in Kegel exercises immediately after delivery may not be suitable for everyone. Postnatal guidance from healthcare professionals can help determine the appropriate time to start and the right intensity for pelvic floor exercises.

Kegel Exercises for Men's Health

Improving Bladder Control: Men can benefit from Kegel exercises to enhance bladder control, especially if they experience urinary incontinence due to various reasons such as prostate issues or surgery.

Erectile Dysfunction: Some studies suggest that Kegel exercises might aid in improving erectile function by enhancing blood flow and strengthening the pelvic floor muscles. However, the efficacy varies among individuals, and consulting a healthcare professional is crucial for tailored advice.

Prostate Health: Kegel exercises can assist in maintaining prostate health by supporting bladder control and potentially reducing the risk of urinary problems associated with prostate conditions.

Proper Guidance: Similar to women, men should perform Kegel exercises correctly to avoid overexertion or strain.

Lifestyle Factors and Pelvic Wellness

Maximizing pelvic health involves considering lifestyle factors, understanding the long-term benefits of consistent Kegel exercises, and employing tips for optimal performance:

Maintain a Healthy Weight: Excess weight can strain the pelvic floor muscles. Maintaining a healthy weight through balanced nutrition and regular exercise can positively impact pelvic health.

Stay Hydrated: Drinking an adequate amount of water maintains bladder health and helps prevent urinary issues.

Healthy Bowel Habits: Avoid constipation and straining during bowel movements, as this can weaken pelvic floor muscles. Ensure a diet rich in fiber and hydration for smoother bowel movements.

Posture Awareness: Proper posture supports pelvic floor health. Avoid prolonged sitting or standing in poor positions that strain the pelvic area.

Avoid Heavy Lifting: Lifting heavy objects improperly can stress the pelvic floor muscles. Use proper lifting techniques and avoid excessive strain.

CHAPTER FOUR

Long-Term Benefits of Consistent Kegels

Improved Bladder Control: Consistent Kegel exercises strengthen pelvic floor muscles, reducing urinary incontinence and improving bladder control over time.

Enhanced Sexual Function: Long-term Kegel practice can enhance sexual sensations, arousal, and orgasm intensity for both men and women.

Pelvic Organ Support: Strong pelvic floor muscles support pelvic organs, reducing the risk of pelvic organ prolapse as individual's age.

Preventative Maintenance: Regular Kegel exercises can help prevent pelvic floor issues, especially for women post-menopause or after childbirth.

Tips for Optimal Kegel Performance

Consistency: Commit to a regular Kegel routine, gradually increasing intensity and duration over time.

Correct Technique: Ensure proper muscle engagement by identifying the right muscles and avoiding tensing other areas like the abdomen or buttocks.

Breathing: Coordinate breathing with exercises; inhale and relax the muscles, exhale and contract them.

Avoid Overexertion: Don't overdo Kegel exercises. Start slowly and gradually increase intensity to prevent muscle fatigue or strain.

Seek Professional Guidance: Consult with a pelvic floor physical therapist or healthcare provider for personalized advice and guidance.

Maximizing pelvic health requires a holistic approach that incorporates healthy lifestyle habits alongside regular and correctly performed Kegel exercises. Consistency, proper technique, and a healthy lifestyle all contribute to achieving and maintaining optimal pelvic floor wellness.

Embracing Kegel Exercises for Lifelong Health

Embracing Kegel exercises as part of your routine can significantly contribute to lifelong pelvic health and overall well-being. These exercises, designed to strengthen and tone the pelvic floor muscles, offer numerous benefits that extend throughout life:

Pelvic Wellness: Kegel exercises promote the strength and resilience of the pelvic floor muscles, supporting bladder and bowel control, as well as the proper positioning of pelvic organs.

Prevention and Management: Consistent practice of Kegels aids in preventing pelvic floor issues such as urinary incontinence, pelvic organ prolapse, and sexual function concerns, particularly after childbirth or with age.

Improved Quality of Life: Strong pelvic floor muscles enhance bladder and bowel control, leading to increased confidence, comfort, and a better quality of life.

Enhanced Sexual Health: For both men and women, regular Kegel exercises can contribute to improved sexual function, sensation, and satisfaction.

Long-Term Benefits: The long-term advantages of incorporating Kegel exercises into daily life include better pelvic support, reduced risk of age-related pelvic issues, and improved overall pelvic health.

By embracing Kegel exercises as a lifelong commitment, supported by proper technique, consistency, and a healthy lifestyle, individuals can proactively maintain and enhance their pelvic health.

Conclusion

Kegel exercises are a valuable and accessible tool for promoting pelvic health and overall well-being. These exercises, aimed at strengthening the pelvic floor muscles, offer a multitude of benefits that extend across various stages of life.

Through consistent practice and proper technique, individuals can:

Enhance Pelvic Health: Strengthening the pelvic floor muscles supports bladder and bowel control, aids in preventing pelvic organ prolapse, and contributes to better sexual health.

Improve Quality of Life: By incorporating Kegel exercises into daily routines, individuals can experience increased confidence, comfort, and improved overall quality of life.

Address Specific Life Needs: Whether during pregnancy, postpartum recovery, or as part of men's health, tailored Kegel exercise routines can address specific health concerns and support long-term wellness.

Embracing Kegel exercises as a lifelong habit, along with considering lifestyle factors and seeking professional guidance when needed, empowers individuals to take proactive steps toward maintaining optimal pelvic health. Consistency, patience, and a holistic approach to pelvic wellness contribute to a healthier and more fulfilling life.

THE END

9 798329 083910